I Can Do It!

I0876994

I Can Stop Germs

By Meg Gaertner

level 1
little blue readers

www.littlebluehousebooks.com

Copyright © 2023 by Little Blue House, Mendota Heights, MN 55120. All rights reserved. No part of this book may be reproduced or utilized in any form or by any means without written permission from the publisher.

Little Blue House is distributed by North Star Editions:
sales@northstareditions.com | 888-417-0195

Produced for Little Blue House by Red Line Editorial.

Photographs ©: Shutterstock Images, cover, 4, 6–7, 8–9, 11, 13, 15 (top), 15 (bottom), 17, 18–19, 21, 22–23, 24 (top left), 24 (top right), 24 (bottom left), 24 (bottom right)

Library of Congress Control Number: 2022901674

ISBN
978-1-64619-579-4 (hardcover)
978-1-64619-606-7 (paperback)
978-1-64619-659-3 (ebook pdf)
978-1-64619-633-3 (hosted ebook)

Printed in the United States of America
Mankato, MN
082022

About the Author

Meg Gaertner enjoys reading, writing, dancing, and being outside. She lives in Minnesota.

Table of Contents

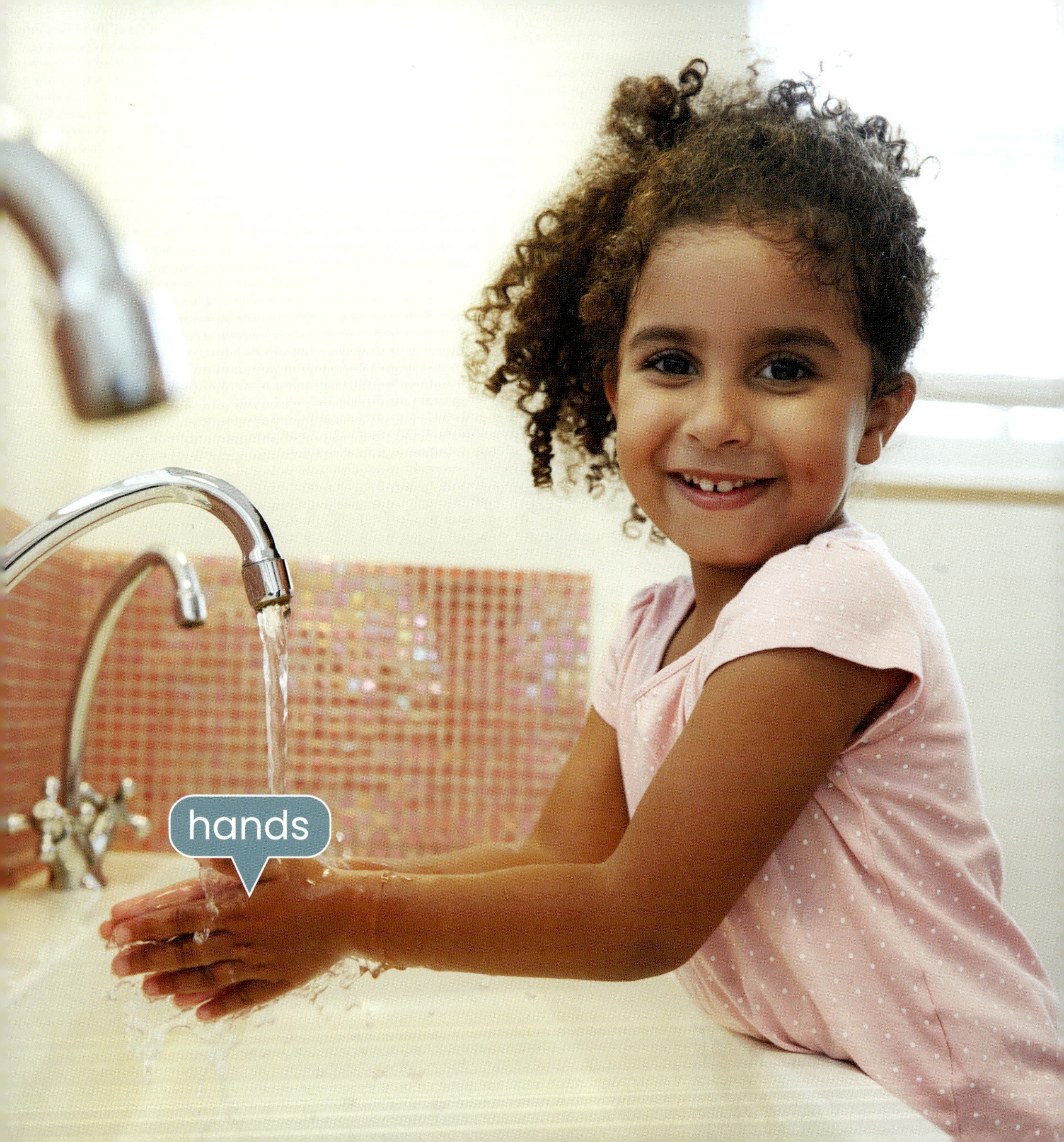
hands

I Can Stop Germs

I can stop germs.

I wash my hands.

I can stop germs.

I use hot water.

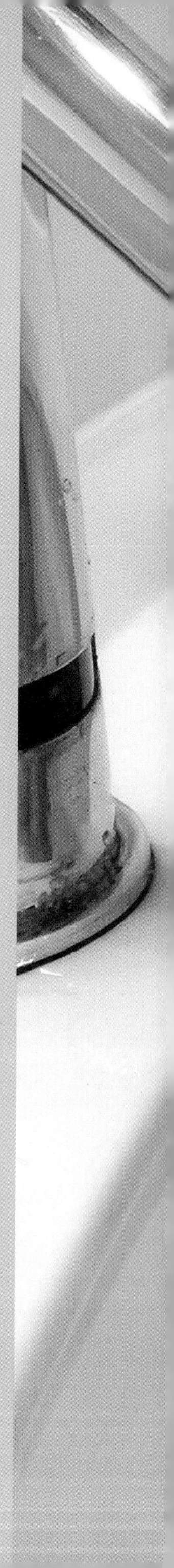

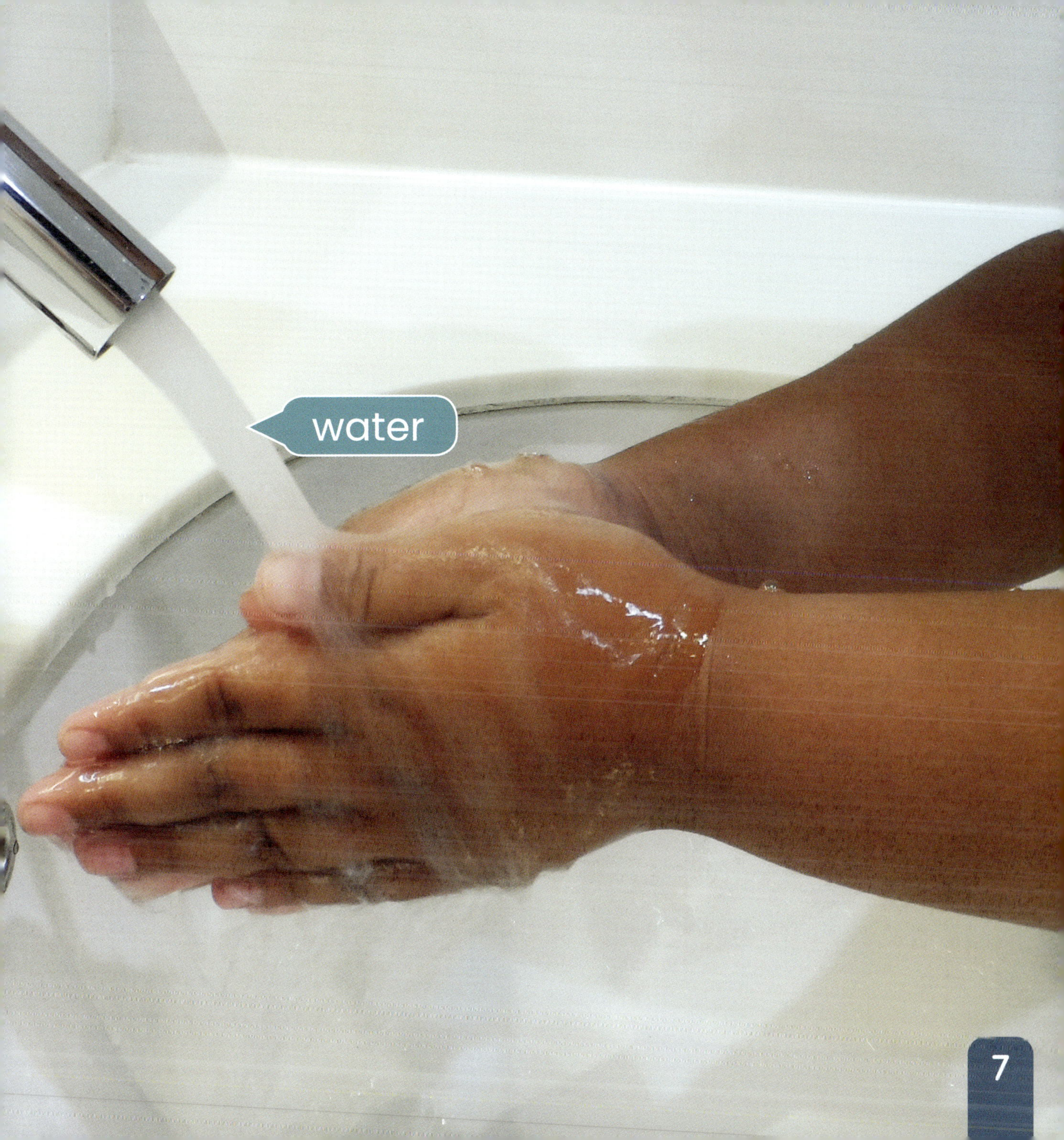
water

I can stop germs.

I use soap.

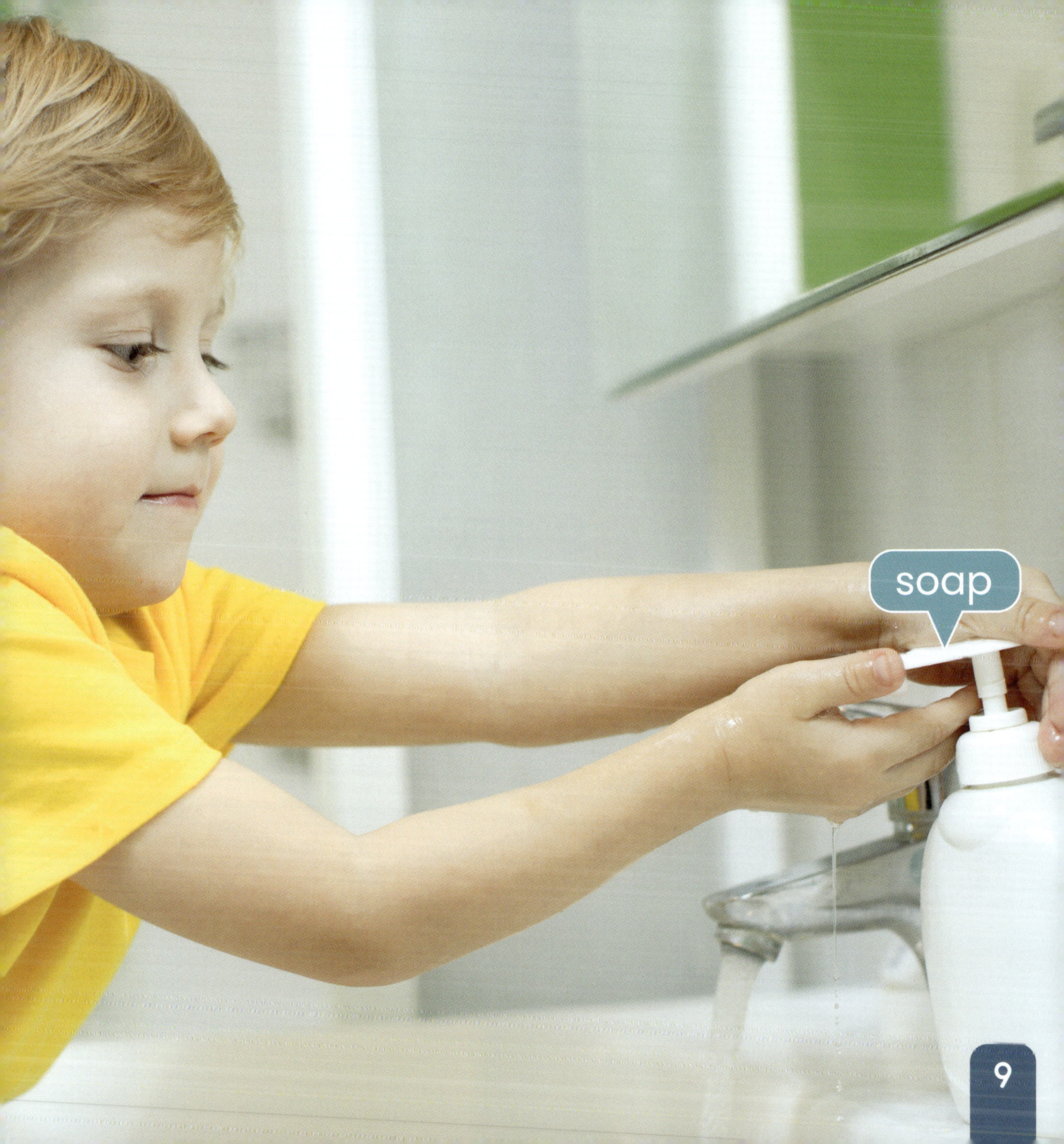
soap

I can stop germs.

I wash my fingers.

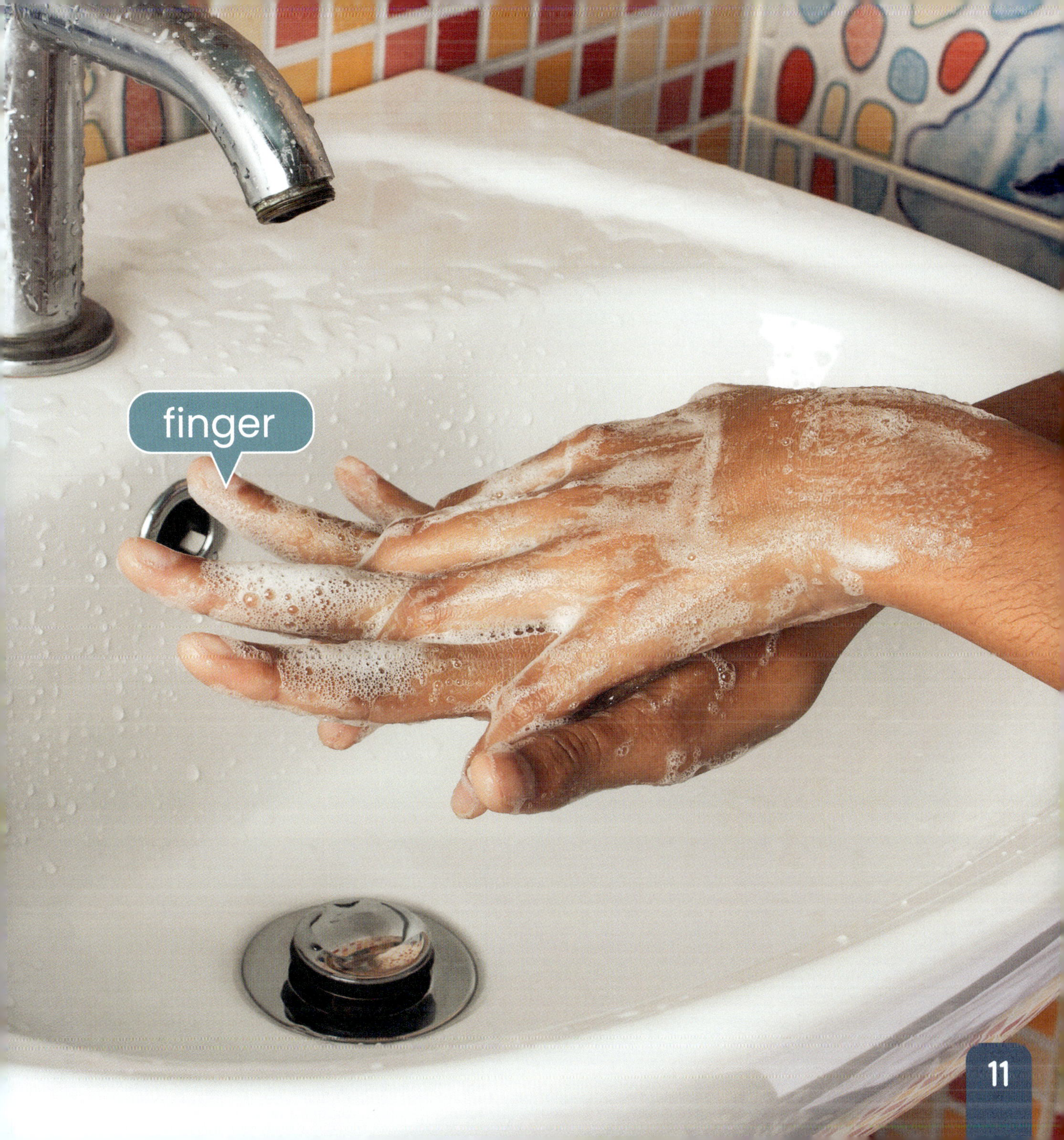
finger

I can stop germs.

I wear a mask.

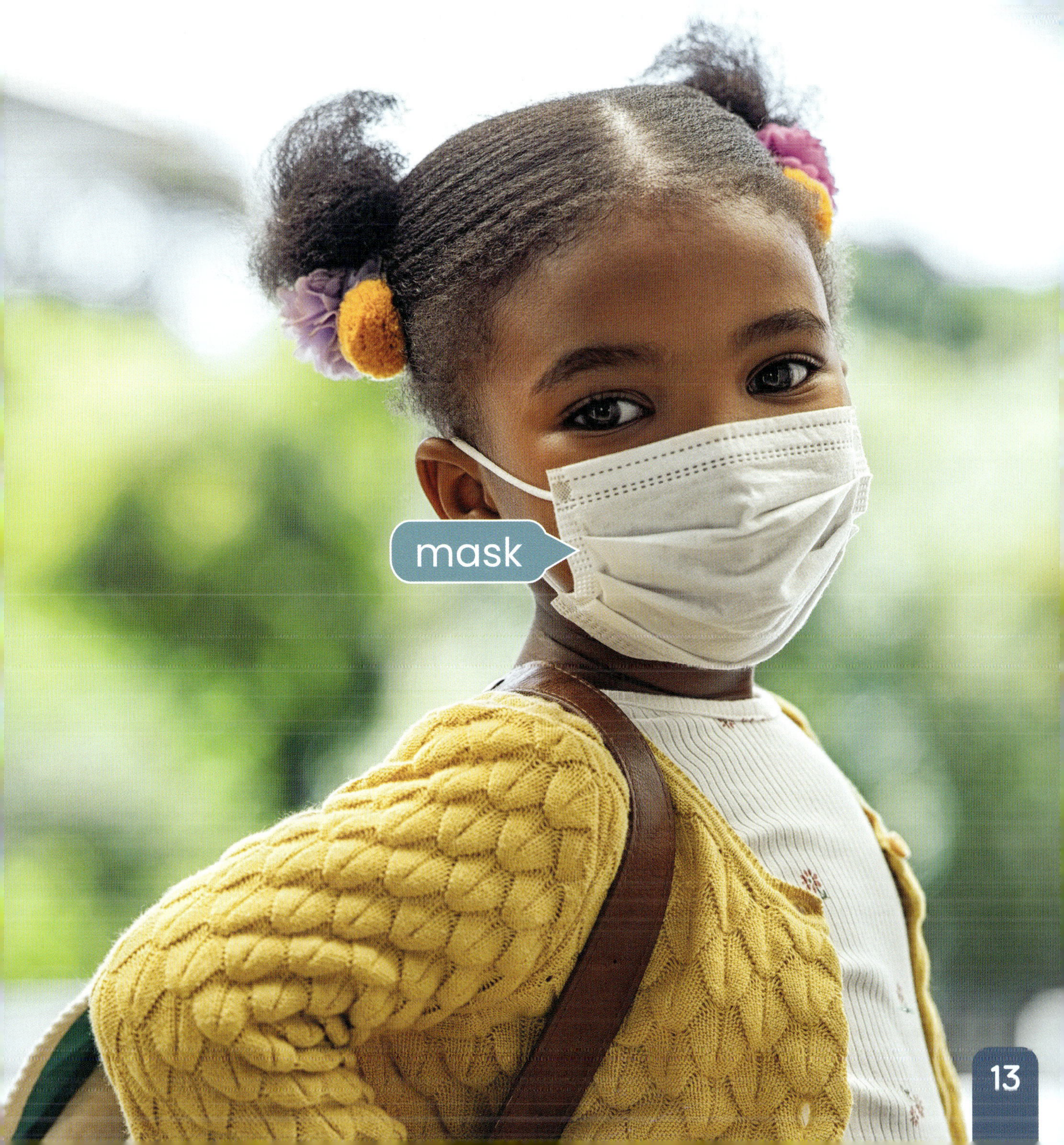
mask

I can stop germs.

I cough into my elbow.

I don't use my hands.

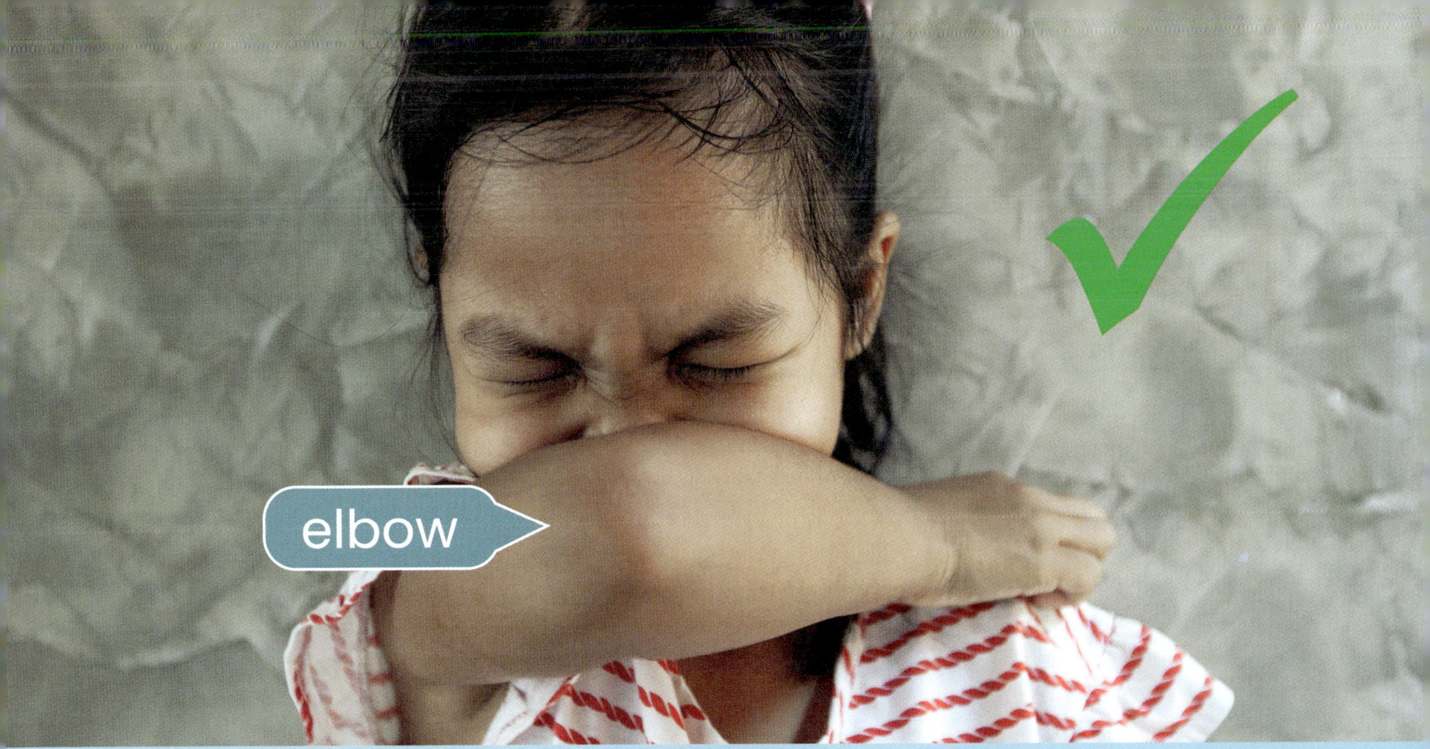
elbow

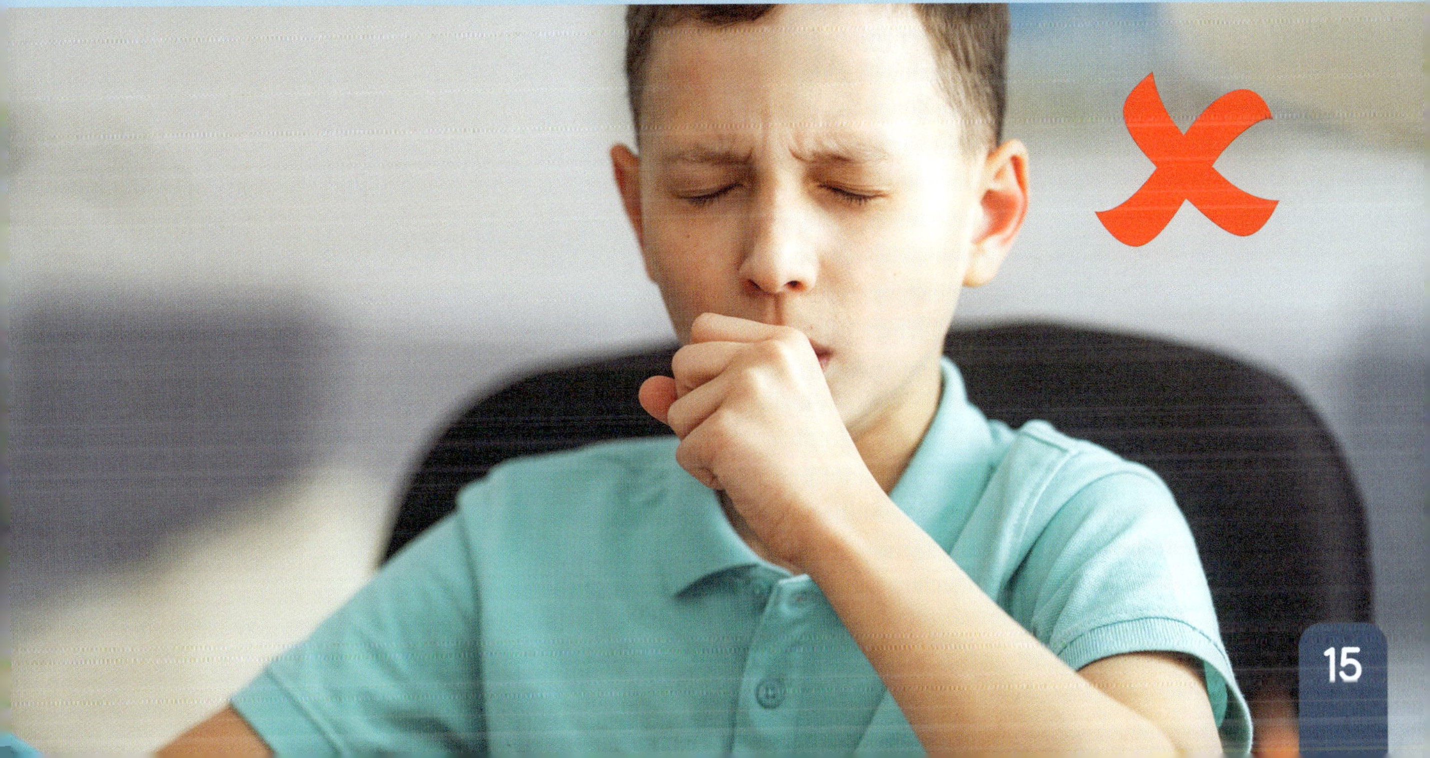

I can stop germs.

I sneeze into a tissue.

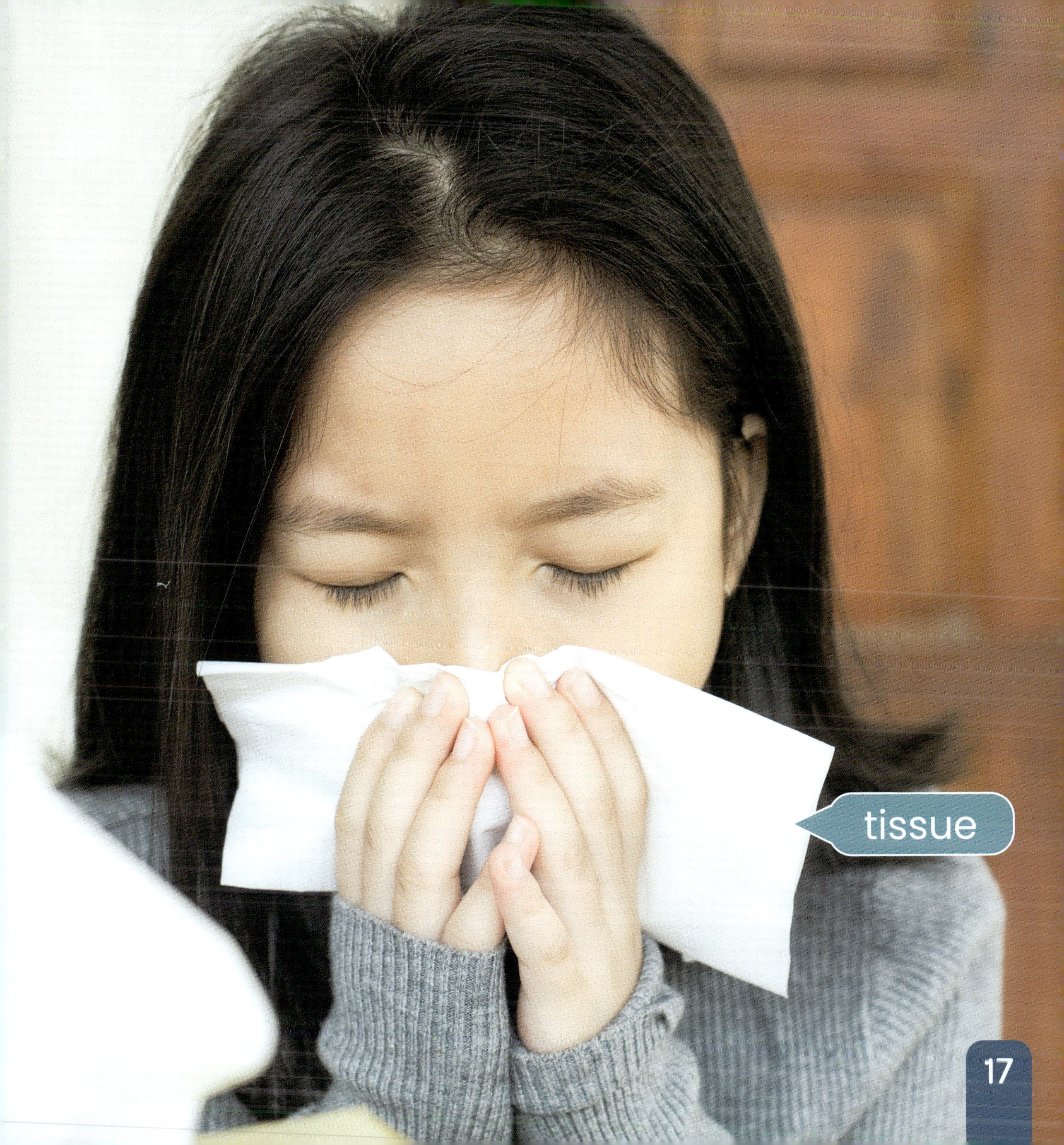
tissue

I can stop germs.

I throw the tissue away.

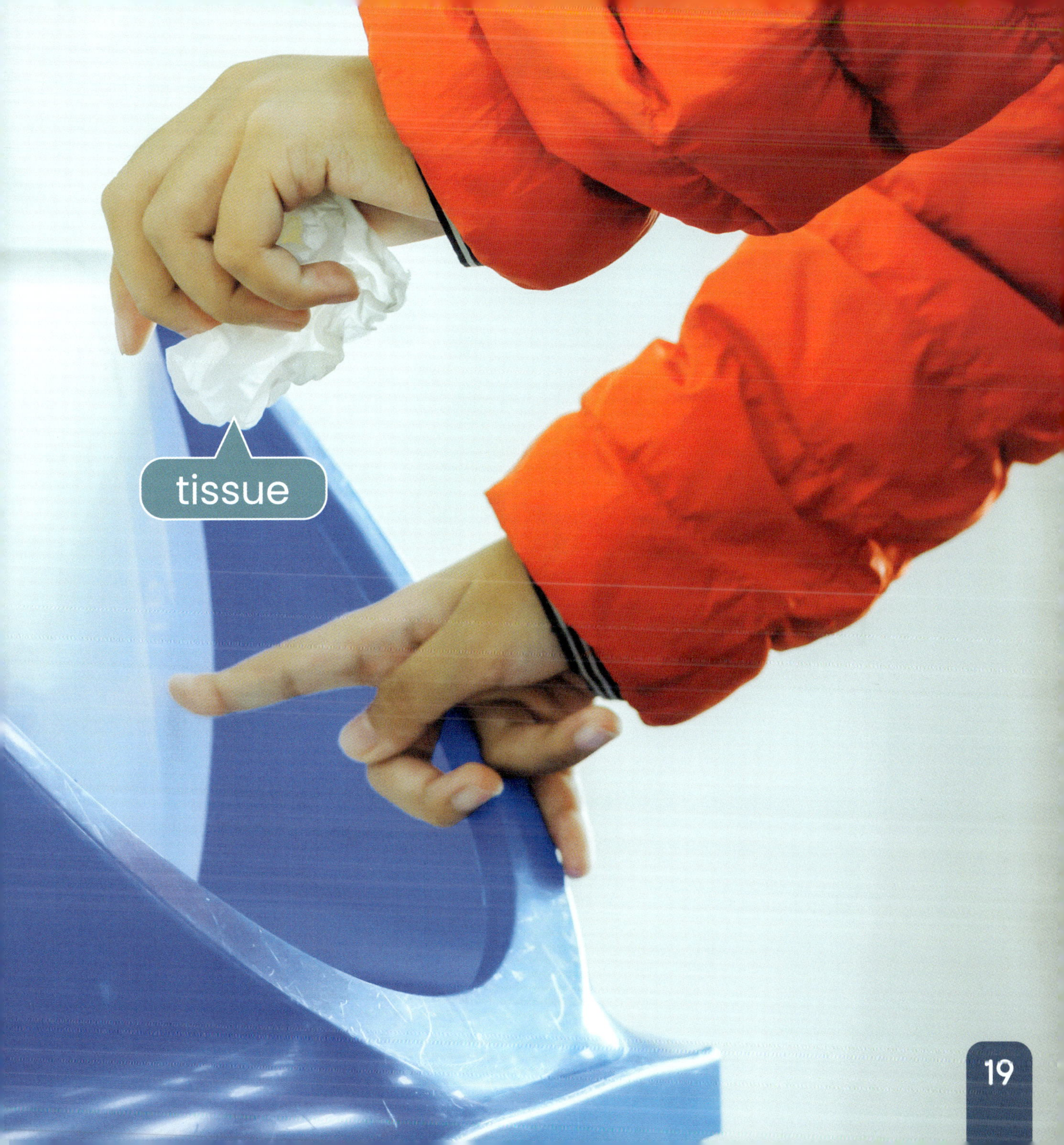
tissue

I can stop germs.

I clean my things.

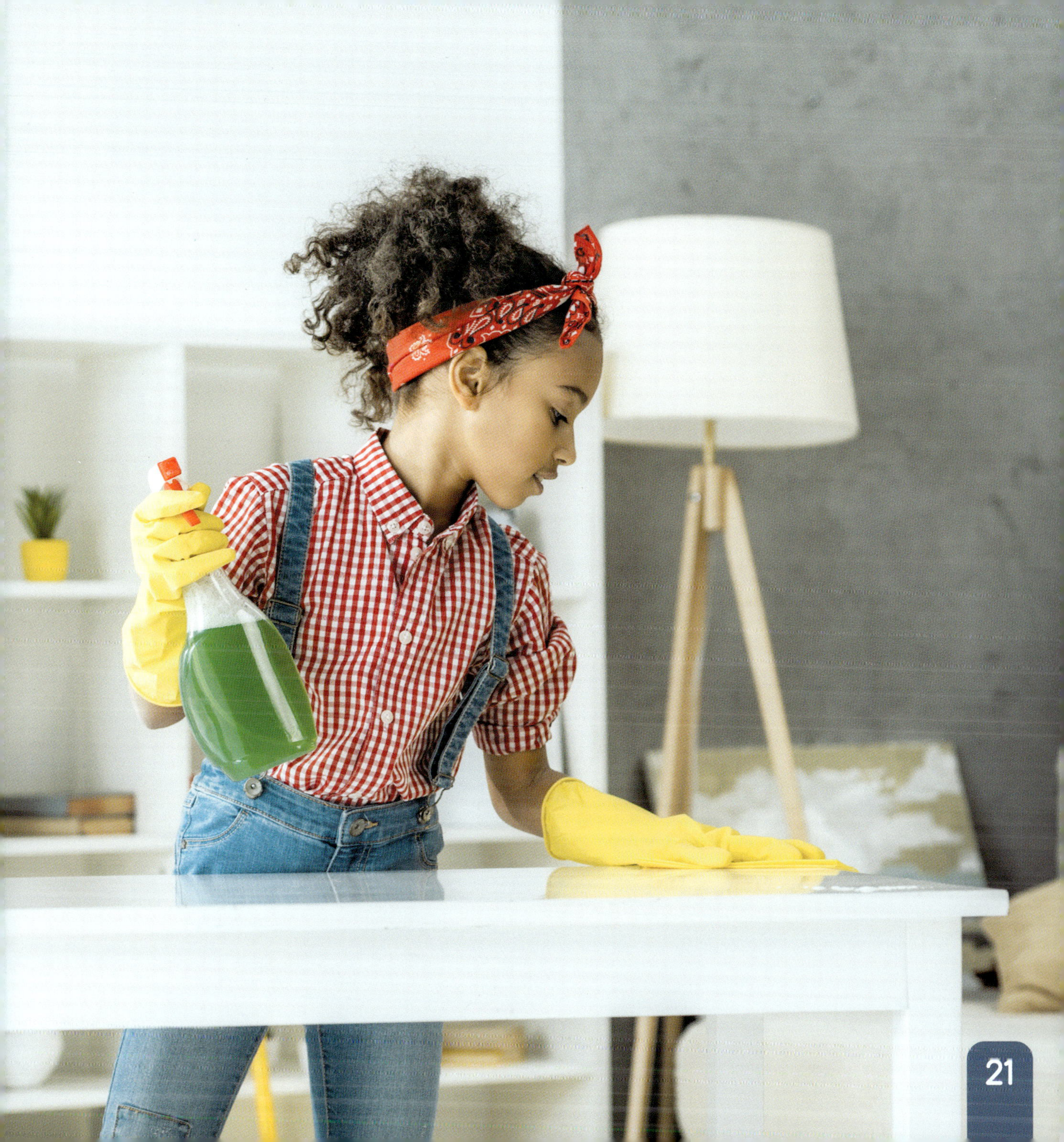

I can stop germs.

I stay home if I'm sick.

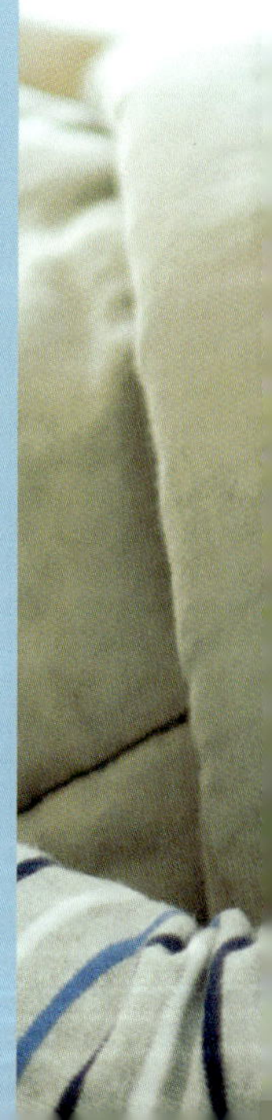

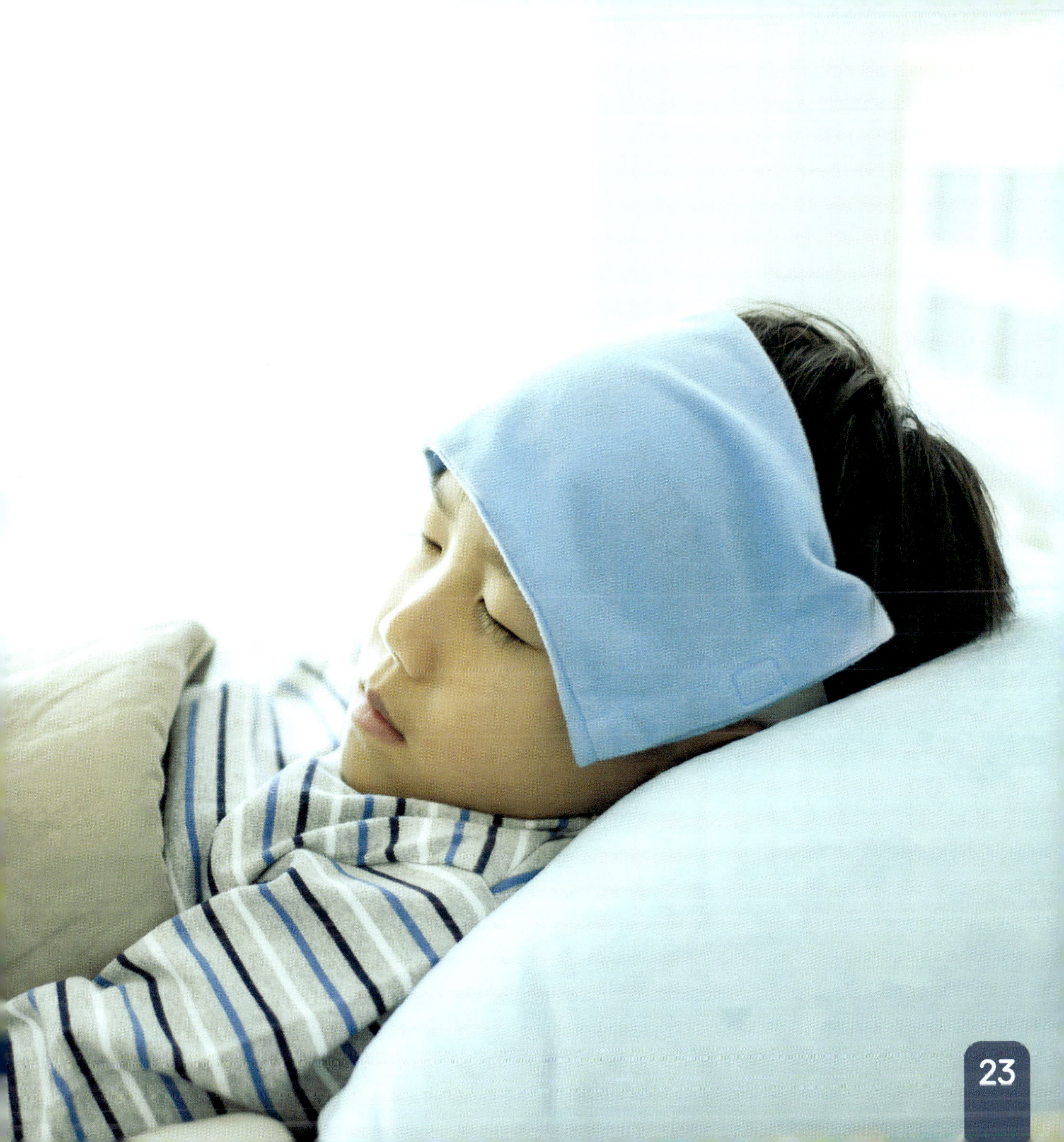

Glossary

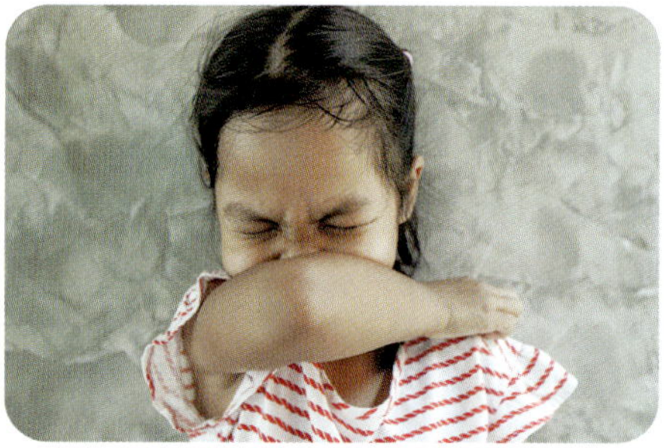

elbow

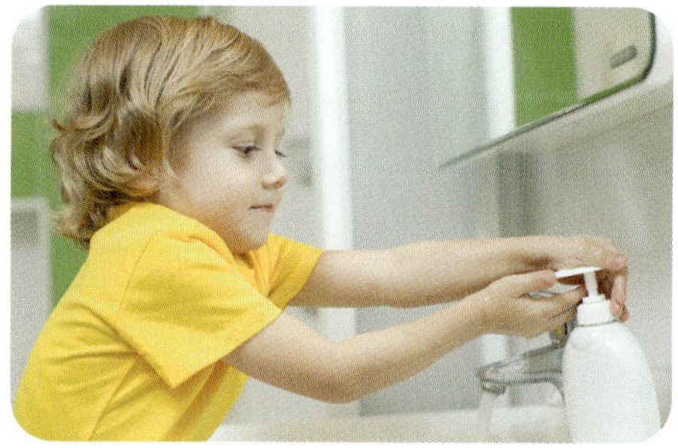

soap

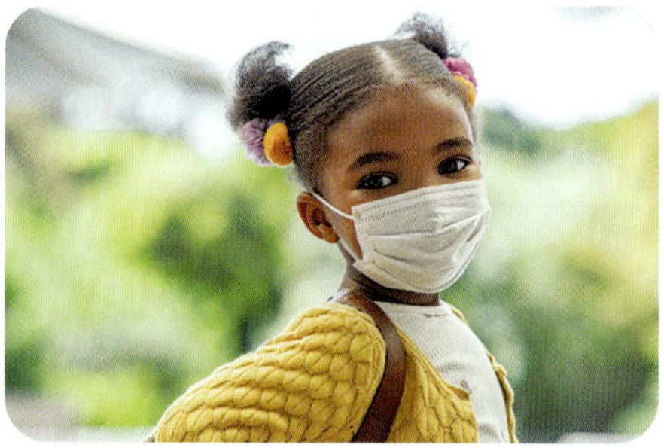

mask

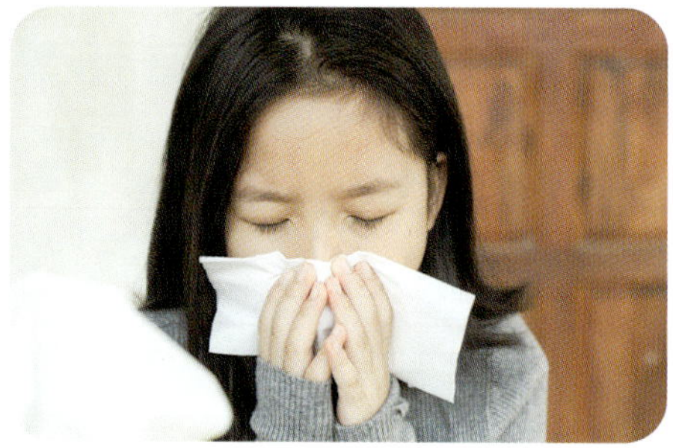

tissue

Index